LITTLE
HEALING BOOK

Daily affirmations to support you
through your cancer healing journey

© 2016 ROSELLA LONGINOTTI

Book illustrations and affirmations by:
Rosella Longinotti - www.rosella-creations.co.uk

Cover design, interior layout and book publishing by:
Chrystel Melhuish - www.plumdesignpublishing.com

Published by Rosella Longinotti in July 2016.
ISBN-13: 978-0-995504103 (paperback)

Disclaimer: This book, its author and the publisher do not make any medical claims, nor is there any suggestion that this book will heal you. The content of this book is about inspiring people and giving emotional support to those who are going through the process.

* The mandala design on the cover is entitled 'Light'

ABOUT ROSELLA LONGINOTTI

I have always considered healing a gift and a vocation. When I began to receive prayers and inspirational words clairaudiently, I knew it was a confirmation of my spiritual path.

Whilst working aboard a ship, I had the opportunity to give a series of creative visualisation meditations and talks on healing. Later, having worked in musical theatre, I became fascinated with using the voice for healing. I found it very powerful and, in 2004, I trained and qualified as a Sound Healer.

The mandalas arrived in 2005, as a psychic bombardment of geometric patterns and an overwhelming compulsion to draw. I began to paint larger mandalas in 2006, and it was not long after that I began to receive the name of the mandala, messages, affirmations and their meanings.

This inspired me to create a set of mandala oracle cards that I use to give insightful readings. I have often been invited to give talks about my mandalas, sharing their messages and their meanings.

Some of my prints can be seen at Akasha Spa, Cafe Royal in London, and in the maternity ward of Russell Halls Hospital in Dudley. I feel that the mandalas encompass all of my gifts in one package, making it easier to share my work.

DEDICATIONS

To my dear friend Leah, who despite being given a diagnosis of seven months to live, lived life with joy and passion for another eight years. Even when sick, she had more energy and zest for life than most people. Leah was an inspiration and always supported and encouraged me to share my healing gifts and inspirational writing with others.

In gratitude to Maud, who came to Mary Le Bow for healing with a brain tumour. When the brain tumour was able to be treated, Maud requested some of my writing to see her through 21 days of radiation treatment. I went home after healing and I wrote what became the nucleus for this book - it just flowed.

In memory of my mother, who was diagnosed with cancer when I was 17 years old and within six months was gone. My first, but not last experience of the sorrow that cancer can bring.

Looking back, I feel that experience sent me in the direction of healing, which was the catalyst for this little book.

'Mothers leave a gap impossible to fill but in time, the pain lessens and you remember only the space they filed with love and not the gap they leave.'

THANK YOU

To Chrystel, for her wonderful enthusiasm, spontaneity and faith in my work, transforming my writing into this beautiful little book.

My dear friend Branka who always gives me lots of support and sound advice.

Josette who has always made time to check my printing projects before they go to print, spotting essential edits and making useful suggestions.

A special thank you to Marilyn for her kindness and support.

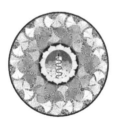

ABOUT THIS BOOK

This small healing book has been created for people undergoing chemotherapy and radiation therapy. The book is divided into four parts:

The first part has affirming messages for the 'Days of Treatment'. These can be read in order or randomly. If you find that you like one especially, you may wish to reflect on it a while longer.

The second part of the book is for the 'Check-up', the third part for the 'Recovery', and the fourth part is for 'Support'.

Each day choose a healing message, read it or say it several times during the day - particularly, when you are feeling anxious. Connect to the healing messages to feel supported.

I hope that this little book blesses you with positivity, and that the gifts of courage, strength and fortitude help you to find peace and serenity within yourself. I wish you well and all the loving support necessary for your healing journey.

Part 1:
AFFIRMATIONS

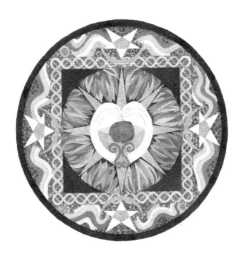

Mandala's meaning: 'Purifying flame
of unconditional love'

Today, I am not a victim
of my sickness.
Although my body may feel
like a battlefield,
I am a warrior
and strength,
perseverance and healing
are my weapons.
My faith creates a vast light over me
and my body and mind
embrace peace.

Today, I release my anxiety,
for I have faith in the doctors
and nurses.
They are doing the best
that they can and have only
my welfare and well-being
as their concern.
I can trust that
through their efforts,
a healing can commence
throughout my body.

Today, the unknown
is known
so my mind
can relax
and I can allow myself
to focus
on the healing
that is taking place
within my body.

Today, I feel more comfortable
in this healing room.
I no longer see it
as a clinical place
but rather as a safe space
where my healing
is taking place.

Today, I am thankful
for all the love
and support
that I am receiving.
I will focus on
that love and kindness,
knowing there are so many
who wish me well.

Today, I am calm,
I know that there is
a divine purpose
to everything
that I experience.
I acknowledge my own
inner spirit,
for that is the key
to my courage
and is the centre
of my calmness.

Today, as the treatment begins
I tell myself:
"Everyone here is
working with me
so that I may be healed.
This is my healing process.
This is the best option for me.
I know healing occurs now
within my body."

I have no anxiety
about today,
I feel relaxed and
have no fear.
Today, I will allow my mind
to think about family
and friends, knowing that
their love surrounds me
and that so many send out
prayers for my well-being.

May I find the healing I need.
May I know peace of mind.
May my heart be serene.
May my body
be free of pain.
May I release
my fears
and anxiety.
May the healing light
shine over me always.

Today, I affirm:
I deserve to be well.
I release the tumour,
the cancer.
I release sickness
and welcome health
into my body.
I deserve to be well.

May I forget
for a moment
the sickness
that rules my life
and live this moment,
this day,
as a well person.

Today, I focus on my breathing.
By breathing deeply,
I can release
any fears
on the 'out' breath
and take in
calm and peace
on the 'in' breath.
I breathe in healing.

Today, I am eager to go
to the hospital/clinic.
There is nothing
to be anxious about,
my faith is strong.
I know the treatment is
fighting disease
so that healing occurs
within me.

Today, I focus on
being a winner
in the battle
that takes place
within my body.
Determination
gives me strength.
I am a warrior.

Today, I feel so strong
that I reassure
everyone else.
I know that healing
is occurring here, now.
I have such a sense
of well-being.

Today, I hold only balance
within me.
The see-saw
of doubts and fears
are stilled.
Today, I trust
in my body's ability
to fight back.

Today, my guardian angel
sits beside me,
hands in mine.
That peace,
that strength
is mine.
Healing flows
through me.

Today, I am free of anxieties.
I will not think
about tomorrow
or "What Ifs..."
I focus only on today,
living each moment
with peace
in my heart.

When I think well of myself,
a stream of golden light
flows through my body
creating a sense of
well-being and healing.

Today, I release hopelessness.
It doesn't belong to me
or with me.
If it attacks me occasionally
then it is unwanted,
for I am full of hope
like a flower bursting
from bud into blossom.
That is my hope.

When love vibrates
from the heart.
The mind is transformed
and is at peace.
Peace of mind
creates a space
for a feeling of well-being.

I release the fear
that sickness
awakens in me.
I release any focus
on 'outcome'.
I release
any pre-meditated thoughts
and attitudes I may have.
I fill the space that remains
with faith and trust
in the healing process.

Today, I release love into my body,
for I lovingly approve of myself.
Love heals my body.
Love heals my mind.
Love heals my emotions.
Love is a healing force
that works within me.

Let faith,
hope and trust
be your words
of affirmation today.
Have faith
in your hopes
and trust
that they will be realised.

Today, I release my fear,
for it is only fear
of the unknown future.
I trust myself
and my strength.

Today, I am filled with peace,
for I know
the healing light
and the prayers
are still streaming my way.
There are so many people
who wish me well
and hold me in their hearts.

Today, I know with certainty
the tumour/cancer is reducing
I have a sense of well-being.
I am halfway through my treatment.
I have infinite faith in all
the healers, doctors and nurses
who help and care for me.

Today, I welcome this moment
of healing treatment,
for I allow my mind to drift
off into the countryside,
and as I breathe in fresh air
and the deep green of nature,
I know that the power of nature
is a healing force
that I can draw upon.

Today, I release my sorrow
and my regrets
and into that space
I pour love
and forgiveness.
Today, I have only peace
within me.

My prayers
are heard
and answered.
There is no fear within me.
Life holds no fears,
for whatever comes my way,
I know now
I have the inner strength.

Today, I release negativity.
I will not expect
the 'worst'.
I accept only the best,
the positive.
Today, I am optimistic,
I know I am improving.

Today, I set aside any stress
I may feel about
what I am experiencing.
I trust the process.
I trust my own ability
to heal.

Healing is more
than a state of mind,
It is a state of being.
We have to want to be well
to the core of our being,
so that every cell
vibrates to that feeling
of well-being.

Still the mind
by being conscious
of the body.
Release any tension.
Relax, breathe deeply.
Slow down,
focus on inner peace,
it can sustain you
when fear threatens
your balance.

Today, I think only positive thoughts
about myself,
and throughout the day
I remind myself,
"I deserve to be well."

Today, I release my doubts.
I replace doubts
with certainty.
I release doubts and
I release sickness.
I welcome healing,
health and balance
back into my life.

Today, I accept the treatment
that I am receiving.
I know it is fighting disease
on my behalf.
The treatment works in harmony
with my body, helping me
with my healing process.

Trust all will be well
and it will be.
Have faith.
You deserve good things
and they will come to you.
Believe you will be healed
and it can be done.

Today, I am alive
and I will celebrate
that I am a survivor.
Today, I celebrate life.
I am a warrior.

Believe in love.
It heals
Love self
it heals.
Love is a river
running through life,
cleansing and healing.
Believe in love.
Love heals.

Don't let fear in.
Yes, that's hard...
But focus always on how far
you've come - the progress.
Now, programme into
your mind and heart
that the spirit within
heals the body -
that miracles do occur and
that you are worthy of them.

I know the treatment is working.
The future is clear -
I am well.
I make plans
for a long
and healthy life.

I greet today with joy,
allowing my mind to drift
off to the seashore.
I am surrounded by the blue
of the sea and sky,
a healing blue,
filling me with peace and calm.
The warmth of the sun upon my body
is re-energising.
The sound of the ocean fills me
with peace and healing.

I am healed by the love that
I feel for myself.
I set aside all self-judgement,
expectations and criticisms.
I allow a loving appreciation
to fill my being.
As I am filled with love,
my body tingles with life
that is a force of healing.

Today, I greet everyone
I see with a smile.
I give encouragement
to those who may need it.
I am thankful that I have
this opportunity to share
for I am so blessed with
those who love and care for me.
My optimism is infectious and
creates a joyous atmosphere.

Today, I set aside
all thoughts
of outcome.
I trust my body's ability
to heal itself.
I have faith in myself.

I am like a diamond
sparkling and bright.
My strength is hard
like a diamond.
My hopes sparkle like diamonds.
The healing force
within me
and over me
is bright like diamonds.

There is a light within me.
It is the light of my spirit.
The spirit within casts
a healing ray
throughout my body.
I am being healed
by the spirit within.
The spirit within,
the me that I am,
works in harmony
with my body.
I allow healing
to begin from within.

Where there is love,
there is healing.
Love has the capacity
to heal all ills,
to repair what is damaged,
to create where there is lack.
What is there to fear or doubt?
Love heals all.

We must have faith
in our body's
ability to heal
if we wish to continue
on the path
of well-being.

We cannot deny
the invasion of sickness,
but we do not have to live
under that shadow of fear
every moment of our day.
Choose life.
Be a warrior.
Believe in miracles and
believe in yourself.
Trust your healing process.

Stay focused
in the 'now' moment.
Feel well now - this moment.
Feel joy now - this moment.
Feel alive and healthy
now this moment.
Be mindful of the moment,
for this is the only moment
that you are living.

Part 2:
CHECK-UP

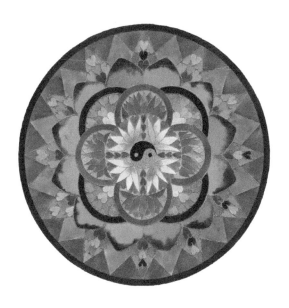

Mandala's meaning: 'Kindness and patience'

I welcome this check-up with joy.
I have no fears or doubts.
This is part of my ongoing
healing process.
I know the doctor wants
only the best for me,
so his/her thoroughness
is for my advantage.
I trust my doctor's words and hands,
and I trust the healing process.
For this check-up is a part
of the caring process.
I have faith that all will be well with me.

The body is a miracle
of creation.
So why not a miracle
of healing?
Trust all will be well
and have faith
in your body.

When all is dark around you,
look within
Open your heart to faith
and trust.
Allow a divine light
to cascade over you,
casting out the darkness,
replenishing your inner light,
so that you are centered
and serene with faith
and trust renewed.

Part 3:
RECOVERY

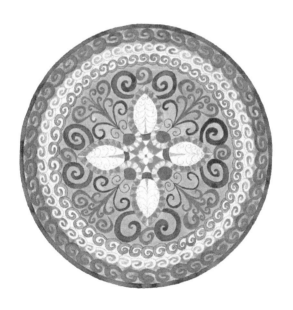

Mandala's meaning: 'Turning over a new leaf'

My body and mind
are at peace,
I deserve this time
of rest and recuperation.
I look forward to
the continuing peace
and healing
that is working within me.
There is balance within me.

I wake each day with a joyful
affirmation of well-being.
I am alive and well.
The day is all mine.
Today, I choose
laughter and happiness,
for both have a positive effect
on my mind and my body.
Today, is a joyous celebration
of being alive.

I begin each day
with a positive thought.
I remind myself today,
that I am special.
I choose to be kind
and patient with myself.
I feel supported by love.
Everyone I talk to today,
confirms, that I hold a special
place in their hearts.

I greet today with joyful optimism,
knowing that my life has been
enriched by my experiences.
I know that I still have goals
I can set for myself.
My life is beginning a new phase,
and I am thankful for this time
where I have this freedom
of choice and the freedom
to experience new things.
Life sends many opportunities,
and I welcome them.
I am thankful that my life
is so blessed.

Today, I am patient with myself.
My body and mind
have been severely tested -
so it is right and proper
that I have time to rest and recover.
I don't have to wake
with the alarm clock,
I can go with the flow.
I make plans for myself.
Life has so much to offer.
Life is a precious gift that I treasure.
I am thankful that I have
this time to myself to create
peace in my surroundings.

Today, I focus on myself.
I set aside any thoughts
about my health
and concentrate
on indulging
my needs.
Today, I embrace life
and enjoy myself.

Pull back the curtains,
open the windows,
breathe in life,
gather up
your enthusiasm.
There is much to be joyous about.
You are alive...
Celebrate life.

Don't give up the fight.
Take time to rest and recuperate.
Allow body and mind
a chance to heal.
Rest and relaxation
are a powerful force
in the healing process.
The treatment has finished,
so the body is in a state
of recovery.
Visualise well-being.

Today, I set aside
time for myself.
I do what I want,
whatever that may be.
For when I know
my own needs,
I am listening
to myself and
honouring myself.

Life is only over
when you give up.
When you tell yourself
that there is nothing
to live or hope for.
But that is a premature thought.
How can life be over when
you are still alive?
Pick up your hopes.
Pick up your dreams and
keep living.

I give thanks that I have this time
to rest my body and mind,
knowing that when all is still,
I am in a state of healing.
I welcome this respite
from work and commitments.
My commitment must be
for my own well-being.
I have time to indulge myself
and my needs.
I am worthy and deserving
of that indulgence.

Today, I allow myself to rest.
I set aside all pressure
to do anything.
I switch off from all the
demands made upon me.
Today, is my day.
I need to rest and recuperate.
I allow myself time to rest and
time for myself.

There is a light over me.
It is the light of healing.
It is never out and never dimmed
for it is the light of God
and when I pray, it shines
even more brightly over me.
It is only my doubts and fears that
create a barrier to this healing light.
So let faith and trust
be my affirmation.
May any doubts I have
be absorbed by that light and
may my healing continue
to manifest God's presence within me.

Today, I have a sense
of freedom and achievement.
I have grown strong
through this experience.
I have discovered
what is important to me.
I am thankful for all the care
that I have been given.
I have no worries or fears
about the future.
I celebrate life with joy
and gratitude.

Part 4:
SUPPORT

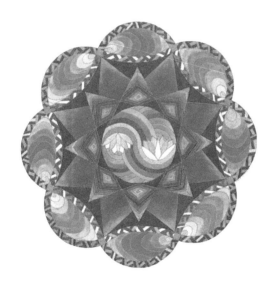

Mandala's meaning: 'Balance flowing like water'

HEALING

The healing light does shine over you.
It is a warm bright light
and it is made up of love,
the love that others bear for you
when they pray or
when they wish you well.
Open to that healing light
feel it and see it.
Let it sustain you
when you are feeling low,
giving you the hope, the courage,
the strength, and of course the healing.

STRENGTH

We have more strength
than we realise,
not perhaps a physical muscular
strength but the infinite enduring
strength that we never knew we had
until we are tested by life's difficulties.
Sometimes we may feel
weighed down by burdens
and think we cannot bear any more.
But somehow we do and that is the
reserve that we never knew we had
and it will forever change us.
For we are so much more
than we ever thought.

LOVE

Love surrounds me
I know.
Each corner
and every area
of my life
is supported
by love.

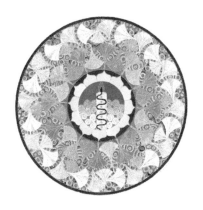

Mandala's meaning: 'Light'

To find out more about Rosella's creative writing, sound healing and beautiful mandalas, visit:
www.rosella-creations.co.uk

Are you a coach, consultant or holistic/spiritual therapist looking to publish your first book or journal for your business? If so, visit:
www.plumdesignpublishing.com/contact
and get in touch quoting LITTLEHEALINGBOOK to get 10% off your first book publishing project.